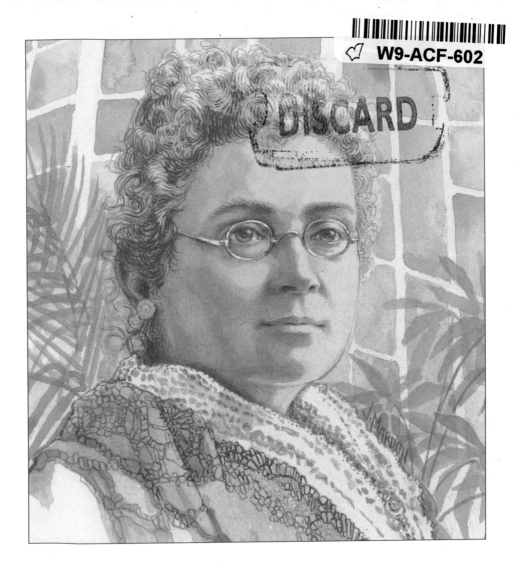

Emily Stowe

Janet Ray

Fitzhenry & Whiteside

Contents

THE CANADIANS
A Continuing Series

Emily Stowe

Author: Janet Ray
Design: Jack Steiner Graphic Design
Cover Illustration: John Mardon

Fitzhenry & Whiteside acknowledge with thanks the Canada Council for the Arts, the Government of Canada through its Book Publishing Industry Development Program, and the Ontario Arts Council for their support of our publishing program.

Canadian Cataloguing in Publication Data
Ray, Janet
Emily Stowe
(Canadians)
Includes bibliographical references and index.
ISBN 1-55041-369-4
1. Stowe, Emily Howard, 1831–1903. 2. Physicians – Canada – Biography. 3. Women physicians – Canada – Biography. I. Title. II. Series.
R464.S76R38 2002   610'.92   C2001-903072-X 2002

© 2002 Fitzhenry & Whiteside Limited
195 Allstate Parkway, Markham, Ontario L3R 4T8

Prologue

O n November 11, 1867, this advertisement appeared in *The Globe*, a Toronto newspaper. Who was this Emily Stowe, calling herself a physician when everyone knew that doctors were always men? She was the first Canadian woman qualified to practise medicine in Canada, and the first entitled to call herself "Doctor." The difficulties she had faced and the obstacles she had overcome to earn that title would have been enough of a challenge to satisfy most people for a lifetime, but not Emily Stowe. Once she had acquired the education and training necessary to qualify as a doctor herself, she set out to make the way easier for other women who would follow her, and to fight the discrimination and blind prejudice that had faced her at every turn.

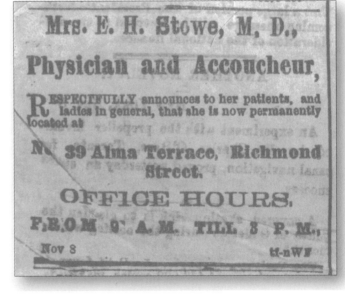

Mrs. E. H. Stowe, M, D.,
Physician and Accoucheur,

RESPECTFULLY announces to her patients, and ladies in general, that she is now permanently located at

No 39 Alma Terrace, Richmond Street.

OFFICE HOURS.

FROM 9 A. M. TILL 3 P. M.,

Nov 3   tf-nWF

Emily Stowe soon realized that women in Canada did not even have the basic rights of citizens and the most basic of these was the right to vote. And so Dr. Emily Howard Stowe helped to start the women's suffrage movement in Canada. The story of this remarkable woman's life began long before she became involved in the field of medicine or in the struggle for the vote. It began in Norwich, Ontario, in 1831.

Chapter 1
The Early Years

On May 1, 1831, a baby girl was born to a very happy Hannah and Solomon Jennings. They named her Emily, and added to this her mother's maiden name, Howard. Emily Howard Jennings was the first of six daughters, followed by Cornelia, Paulina, Hannah Augusta, Ethlinda and Ella. The family lived in the village of Norwich about thirty-two kilometres southwest of Brantford. It was in this small community that the six girls grew up and developed the strong beliefs that were to be so important in Emily's life.

Hannah and Solomon Jennings were Methodists, but they had originally been Quakers. This Quaker background had a very strong influence on the young Emily, because the Quakers believed that a good education was vitally important for everyone. They also believed that women were equal to men. Emily was sure to have a thorough education, not just one that had been watered down for girls. She would learn more than the usual homemaking skills designed to make girls efficient mothers and wives.

Also because of her Quaker background, Emily was not brought up to have any doubts about her own abilities and intelligence simply because she was a girl. Instead she learned that girls were as capable as boys and were expected to shoulder their share of responsibilities as well as rights in the home and in the church. Women were equal partners with men.

In the mid-1800s Norwich was still a pioneer community and everyday life was hard by our standards. Emily learned very early that a person had to be strong and competent even to do such tasks as preparing meals, keeping a house clean and comfortable, providing food and clothing for a family, or travelling to neighbours' homes or to other parts of the country. When Emily was a child there was no indoor plumbing, no electric lights, stoves, or other electric appliances to make work easy.

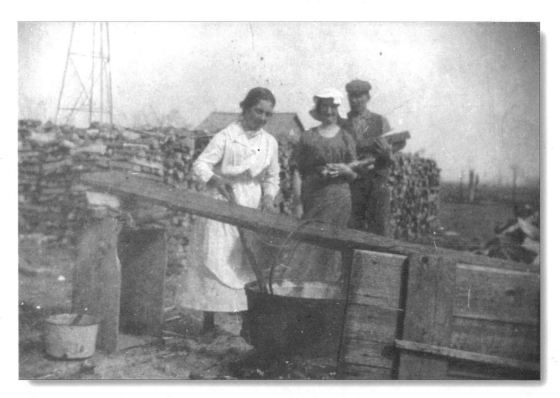

Such everyday tasks as doing the family wash demanded a good deal of time and effort. Many women still made their own soap, which was a long and complicated process. The family would collect hardwood ashes to make lye, and carefully store away the grease and fat from cooking until there was enough to boil with the lye in huge outdoor vats. Sometimes fine sand was added to give the soap extra scrubbing power. The mixture was then poured into moulds to harden.

Even for women who did not make their own soap, washday was hard work. The water had to be boiled and poured into huge tubs—one for soaking the clothes, one for blueing, another for scrubbing and a last for rinsing. The actual washing demanded considerable physical strength since clothes had to be thoroughly scrubbed up and down on a washboard. By mid-century there were washing machines of a kind, but these made the task of scrubbing and wringing the clothes only a little easier. In addition, the machines were so unreliable that at times they were more bother than they were worth. Clothes were hung out on a line to dry. This became a real problem in winter because

Soap making was common in many rural areas even into the twentieth century

the clothes quickly froze into stiff, awkward shapes that had to be wrestled off the line.

The clothes which took so much time and effort to wash had all been made at home. With a large family like the Jennings, all of whose clothes were sewn at home; the task was enormous. Even the simplest wardrobe for each person included night clothes and underclothes as well as many layers of outer garments for both winter and summer. All the children had to help make the clothes, and at a very early age both boys and girls were skilled at knitting such items as undershirts.

The only way to travel in those days was by horse and buggy, or, in the winter, by horse and sleigh. This was much less romantic than it sounds because the passengers were exposed to all kinds of weather and the roads were frequently no more than dirt tracks. The only other way of getting from one place to the next was by walking. There were few railroads in Canada at that time.

The horse and buggy was the usual way of travelling

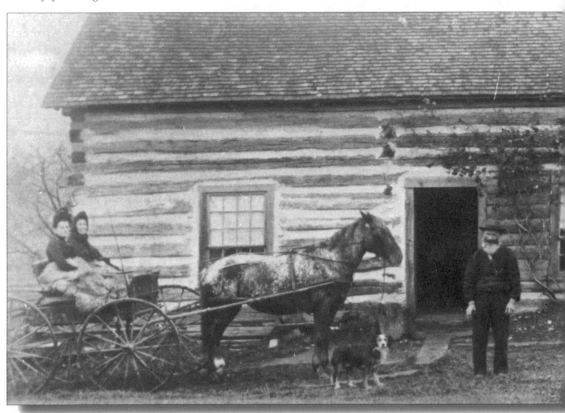

The Early Years

There were not even many schools, particularly in rural areas. Although the idea of no schooling may sound appealing, a lack of education was a serious handicap for many people. In the larger cities there were more schools but they were mainly for boys. The few girls' schools usually concentrated on teaching subjects like French, singing and needlepoint. Since girls were expected to become wives and mothers, they were given only those lessons that were supposed to help them fill these roles graciously and skillfully. Little or no thought was given to preparing them for careers, or even for earning a living. Their husbands would look after that. Because of this, women who did not marry or were widowed were usually little prepared to take care of themselves.

Partly because of her parents' Quaker background, Emily did not find herself in such a situation. Also, Hannah Jennings's interest in education went back a long way. Her grandfather had opened the first school in Norwich in his own

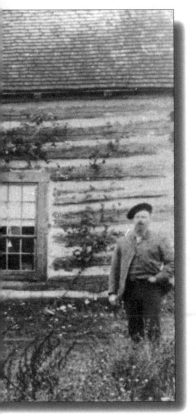

house. Hannah knew how important an education was, so to make sure that her six daughters had a complete schooling, she taught them herself. Emily was so good a pupil that at the age of fifteen she was teaching school herself.

Chapter 2
The Young Teacher

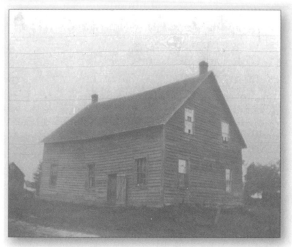

An example of an early one-room schoolhouse

Emily began her teaching career in a small rural school near the town of Norwich. It was a plain, wooden framed building with a single classroom. As the only teacher, she was responsible for all grade levels. This meant that when she prepared a lesson for one grade, she also had to arrange assignments and exercises to keep the other children occupied. It was no easy task to make sure everyone was learning something.

Her evenings were spent preparing lessons so that the next day while she was reviewing spelling with Grade 1, Grade 2 students would have a story to read, Grade 3 would be drawing maps, and so on. Part of the problem with teaching was that the students could keep no record of what they had learned. They usually did their assignments in chalk on small slate boards. When the exercise was finished, the slate was wiped clean, ready to be used again. Emily had to be sure that her students had really learned the information on their slates before they wiped it away.

Another problem she had was that many pupils did not attend school very regularly. In the mid-1800s, children were expected to help out with the family's work. If there was work to be done around the house, on the farm, or in the shop, the boys and girls did not go to school until the jobs were done. Then they would reappear in Emily's classroom and it would be up to her to help them continue their education.

Besides preparing lessons and teaching all the different grades, teachers were usually responsible for keeping the school clean and tidy. After classes were over, Emily had to

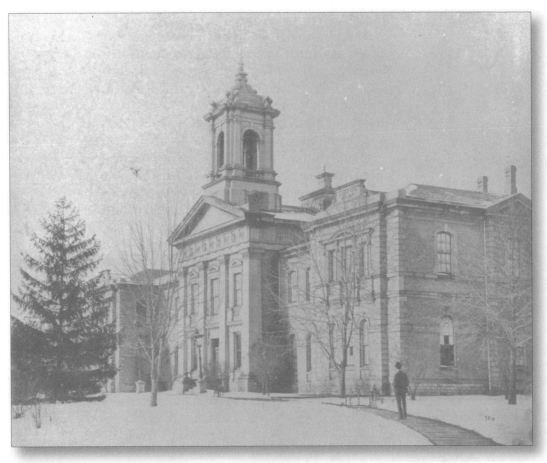

The Normal School in Toronto

clean and sweep the rooms, take out the garbage and, in winter, keep the fire in the stove going to heat the school.

Despite the great amount of work involved in teaching in a rural school, Emily liked the job. She enjoyed the challenge of opening the doors to knowledge through teaching the "three R's"—reading, 'riting and 'rithmetic. Emily was a good teacher, probably because she herself took such pleasure in learning. After a few years of teaching, she wanted to improve her own education, so when she was in her early twenties, Emily made up her mind to go to university.

This was easier said than done. Her family gave her support and encouragement because they believed that education was important, but the universities at the time did not admit women. Emily must have known this, but she applied anyway

The Young Teacher

to the University of Toronto. She thought it was silly that they would refuse a good student simply because she was a woman and she knew that she had the ability for university courses. Nevertheless her application was turned down. This setback was very disheartening, but Emily was determined. She decided that the only thing she could do was to continue teaching and save as much money as possible so that she could at least go to the Normal School in Toronto.

Going to the Normal School meant that she would learn more about teaching, but she would also be able to find a better teaching position and get a better salary. Emily worked very hard during the year she spent at the school. There was much to learn and many hours of studying to do because she wanted to graduate with a high standing, but she had not really expected to do as well as she did. When she graduated from the Normal School for Upper Canada in 1854, she had earned a First Class Teacher's Certificate. Much to her surprise, the Brantford School Board offered her the position of principal at the Brantford public school. Emily accepted and became the first woman principal in Canada.

This was a challenging and exciting time in Emily's life. She was a part of the teaching profession just at a time when education in Ontario was changing and improving. Much of this change was because of the influence of one man, Egerton Ryerson. In 1844 he had been appointed Superintendent of Education in Upper Canada, and it was his plan that every child should have an equally good chance to get an education.

Before this, especially in rural areas, children might not get an education unless their parents joined together to hire a teacher and provide a school. But pressure had been put on the government to take a hand in the education of the young, and finally the Common School Acts had been passed in

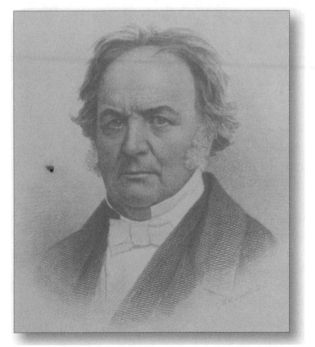

Egerton Ryerson

1846, 1847 and 1850, so everyone had the right to a free education. In fact, by 1871 it was more than a right; attending school was compulsory, but for only four months of ever year, and then only for students between the ages of seven and twelve.

Although education was generally improving in Ontario, teachers' salaries were low. By 1850 a large number of women had gone into teaching, and many school boards hired them instead of men because they could pay women teachers half the salary they would have to pay men. In the Toronto Common School System in 1858, the salaries for men, depending on their rank, ranged from $520 to $700 a year. Women teachers, on the other hand, earned between $170 and $400 a year. This seems very unfair when both the men and women had taken the same amount of training and taught the same grades. One of the reasons given for such a difference in pay was that men had a family to support, while women had only themselves to look after. Women were expected to marry at some time and leave teaching to raise a family. Then their husbands would support them and they would not need to receive as much pay as men. This was not really a good argument since some women never married, and some, like Emily, found that women too had to support families on these low salaries.

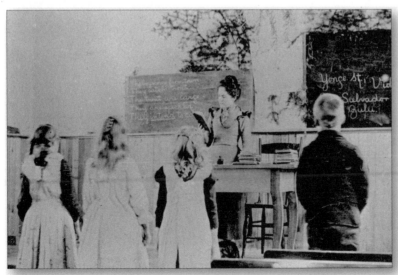

Ontario schoolroom in the 1880s

Chapter 3
A Time for Decision

W hen Emily went to Brantford to take up her new position as principal, more changed in her life than just her job. Most of that change was caused by a young man named John Stowe.

John was from Mount Pleasant, a small town about eight kilometres southwest of Brantford. He had been born in Yorkshire, England, and, at the age of thirteen, had come with his family to Canada. The family settled in Mount Pleasant and John's father built an octagonal house that had a wagon shop and blacksmith shop on the ground floor and living

Central High School in Brantford, where Emily Stowe was principal

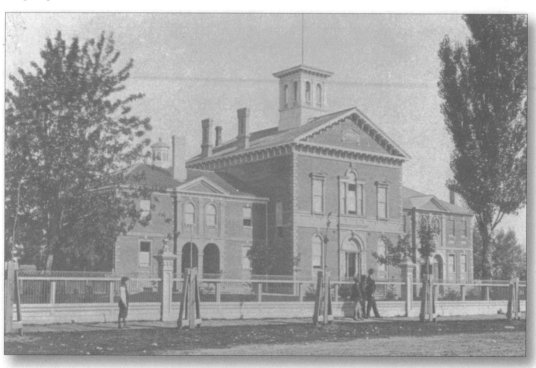

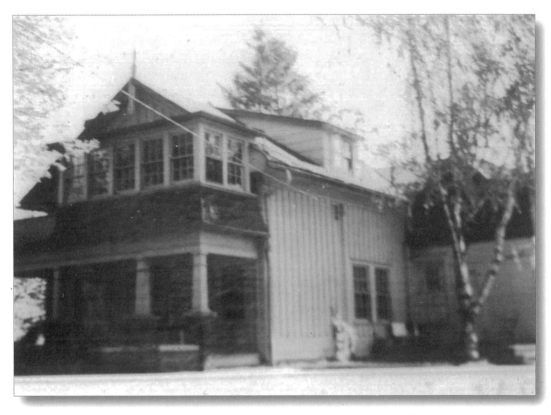

The Stowe home in Mount Pleasant, built by John Stowe

quarters upstairs. There John spent his adolescent years and learned his father's craft. By the time he was courting Emily, John was working as a carriagemaker.

In 1856 Emily Jennings and John Stowe were married and Emily left the teaching profession to become a homemaker. With the help of his brother William, John built another octagonal house in Mount Pleasant for himself and Emily, and they settled down to raise a family.

These were very happy times, made even happier over the next few years by the births of three children. Augusta came first, in July, 1857. Then in February, 1861, Augusta's first brother, John Howard, was born, and Frank Jennings arrived two years later in February, 1863.

For several years the Stowe family prospered. The three children played with friends, helped their parents about the house, and attended school when they were old enough. Among their very close friends were the children of the Nelles family who lived across the street. Dr. William Waggoner Nelles ran a school, and it is likely that John Stowe built the Nelles Academy, for it, too, was an octagonal building.

Emily's life was busy and full, looking after her husband, caring for her children, and visiting with friends. She had always thought that the role of wife and mother was very important, and she felt that women could make a great contribution to Canada by providing good, loving homes. Much later, in 1889, she said,

I believe homemaking, of all the occupations that fall to woman's lot, [is] the one most important and far reaching in its effects upon humanity...

But for Emily the role of mother and homemaker was not to last very long. John's health had been failing for some time and finally the doctors said he had tuberculosis. This meant he would have to enter a sanatorium in order to regain his health. Emily realized that she would have to return to teaching to support the family and pay the medical bills. When their friend Dr. Nelles offered her a position at his academy, she quickly accepted. At least she would not have to travel far and would always be close to her children.

It must have been very hard for Emily to raise her family on the low salary that women teachers were given, but she did it. She also made a decision that would make her life even more difficult, for it was while her husband was in the sanatorium that she resolved to become a doctor.

It may have been partly John's illness that made Emily want to become a doctor, but she had also been aware for a long time of the great need for women doctors. Women would often go for years bearing the pain and inconvenience of infections and ailments because they were too modest and shy to go to a male doctor. There were many times when a minor problem would develop into a serious illness just because a woman did not want a male doctor to look after her. Emily thought that this was completely wrong. All that was needed was some women doctors who would understand women and their ailments.

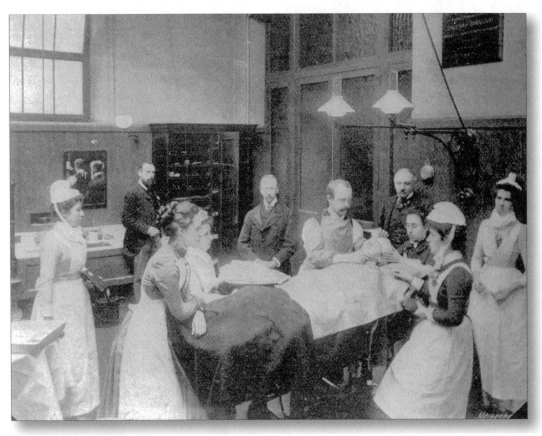

Performing an operation in the late 1800s

To train as a doctor, Emily had to save enough money to pay for her training and to support her family at the same time. She carefully saved all she could from her teaching salary at the Nelles Academy. Even so, it meant that all the members of the family had to do their part to help. While all the bills were paid and food and clothing were provided, they could afford few luxuries. Life was hard, and Emily had to work long hours as well as look after her three children. One reason she was able to carry such a load was that her family helped; another was that she was determined to become a doctor. When Emily had set her mind on something, nothing would stop her.

Chapter 4
Another First

Emily soon found that she needed more than just determination to become a doctor. Before she could even enter medical school, she had to return to studying. Applicants for university had to pass college entrance examinations. Her life during the months of preparation for the exams was hectic and exhausting. Every day, before going out to teach at the Nelles Academy, Emily had to get the children up, give them breakfast and send them off to school. After the day's work, there were meals to be cooked, clothes to be sewn and washed, and the house to be kept clean. In the evening, Emily prepared lessons for the next day's classes, and when this was done, she had to start on long hours of study for her examinations.

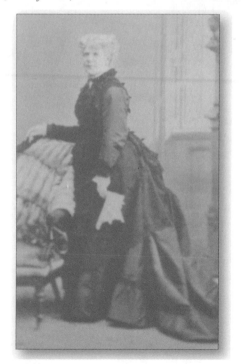

Emily's sister, Cornelia

Fortunately, she received some help. Emily's sister, Cornelia, offered to care for the children while John was in the sanatorium and Emily was teaching. Augusta, Frank and John were very fond of Aunt Cornelia, who was often a substitute mother for them. Cornelia later married Judge Drew R. Tilden and went to live with him in Cleveland, Ohio. Still later she travelled about Europe, dressed in the modest outfit of a Quaker, collecting items for an American gallery. Like her sister, she was quite a remarkable woman.

With the help of Cornelia and the support of her family, Emily succeeded in looking after the family needs and in saving enough money for her training. The next step was to apply to a university. Because it was fairly close to her home and had a very good reputation, Emily chose the University of Toronto and applied

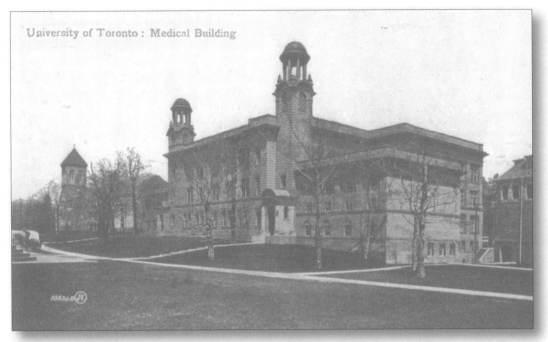

University of Toronto Medical Building

for admission to its medical school. After waiting anxiously for what seemed like a very long time, the answer from the university finally arrived. Her application had been refused. The only reason was that she was a woman, and the authorities felt that women students would make discipline too difficult.

Although Emily was bitterly disappointed by the verdict of the university, she was not surprised. At this time it was generally thought that a woman's place was in the home and the only role a woman should play was that of wife and mother. If a woman had to work to support either herself or her family, there were very few respectable occupations open to her. Only recently had women been accepted as teachers.

A woman could enter domestic service or do sewing in a shop or at home, both at unbelievably low wages and neither very appealing. In the 1860s, nursing was disorganized and was not yet considered a suitable occupation for most women. Nurses in some hospitals were dedicated members of religious orders, but in most hospitals the nurses were slovenly and had had little, if any, training. In England, Florence Nightingale was beginning to organize schools to train nurses, but nursing schools were not established in Canada for some time.

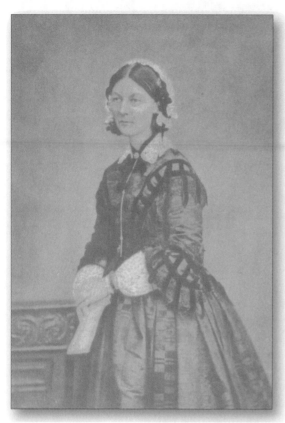
Florence Nightingale

The other professions such as medicine, law, or even a career in politics were thought to be far too demanding and, even more important, too coarse for women. Women were thought to be so delicate that they would not have the physical or mental strength to deal with the challenges of these careers. People forgot that bearing children and caring for a home in the nineteenth century took as much, if not more, strength than any of the professions.

So when Emily Stowe applied for permission to study to become a doctor, she was fighting against deeply rooted public opinion. The only people not shocked at her decision were her family. Their Quaker background and beliefs had given Emily her faith in herself and in the ability of women.

In the United States the situation was not quite as bad as in Canada. The way had been opened up by Elizabeth Blackwell who had graduated from the Geneva Medical College in New York State. She had been rejected by dozens of medical schools and the authorities of the Geneva Medical College agreed to admit her only if every one of the male students voted to accept her. Some of the students saw it as a good joke and others thought women should be doctors, so they all voted for her and Elizabeth began her training. But after she graduated in 1849, the college ruled that no more women would be admitted.

If the other schools of medicine would not allow women to have an equal chance with men, then the answer was to create new schools. Dr. Elizabeth Blackwell worked to raise support and money for a medical school so that other women would be able to become doctors. Eventually she founded the Woman's Medical College of the New York Infirmary for Women and Children. The Quakers of Philadelphia also felt that there was a great need for women doctors. They helped to establish the

Another First

Woman's Medical College of Pennsylvania in 1850. Yet another medical school for women was founded by Dr. Clemence Sophia Lozier. In 1863 she opened the New York Medical College for Women. It was this college that Emily attended to train as a doctor, since no college in Canada would accept her.

While Emily was away studying in New York, Aunt Cornelia stayed in the Stowe home in Mount Pleasant to look after the family. The children missed their mother, and the reason for her absence also made Augusta, John and Frank feel different from their friends. Some children had mothers who worked to help the family, but none of them had a mother who wanted to be a doctor. It was sometimes hard to have a father who was only slowly recovering his health and a mother away at medical school.

Finally in 1867, the same year that Canada achieved Confederation, Emily Stowe succeeded in her deepest desire and graduated as a doctor. Much to her family's delight, she returned to Canada, collected them all from Mount Pleasant and moved to Toronto. There she opened her office at 39 Alma Terrace on Richmond Street, and became the first Canadian woman to practise medicine in Canada.

There had actually been another woman doctor in Canada before Emily. Dr. James Miranda Stuart Barry had practised medicine in Canada in the 1850s. But she was British, and had spent only a few years in this country as Inspector-General of Hospitals in Upper and Lower Canada. She got that position by disguising herself as a man, which she did throughout her life so that she could be a British Army medical officer.

Chapter 5
In Practice

E ven after she had graduated as a doctor and had set up her practice in Toronto, Emily's difficulties were not over. There was still another barrier she had to overcome to establish herself in her chosen profession, and it was a problem that she had not expected. Shortly after she had graduated from the New York Medical College for Women and returned to Canada, an Act of Parliament was passed. According to this Act, all doctors who had trained in the United States had to take a matriculation examination before a Council of the College of Physicians and Surgeons of Ontario in order to get a licence to practise medicine. They also had to attend at least one session of lectures at an Ontario medical school.

King Street, Toronto, in the late 1860s

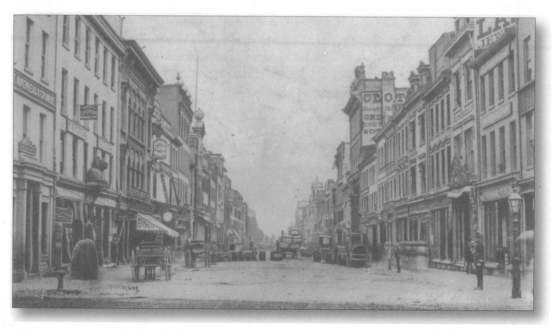

In Practice

This law was passed to make sure that doctors who had trained outside Canada met Canadian medical standards. The obvious problem for Emily was that no Ontario medical school would admit women, and the College of Physicians and Surgeons would not license a doctor who had not met this requirement. There was also a fine of one hundred dollars for practising medicine without a licence. It was impossible and preposterous, but there was no way out of the dilemma. So, despite the fines, Emily went ahead and practised without a licence until she could find a solution. For one reason and another, that was to take thirteen years.

Although Emily regularly and persistently applied to the University of Toronto to be admitted to the Medical School, the university just as regularly refused to admit women, even for one session. After receiving one of the many refusals, Emily replied with hope and defiance:

Your Senate may refuse to admit women now, but the day will come when these doors will swing wide open to every female who chooses to apply.

Third-year students at the University of Toronto Medical School, 1870–71

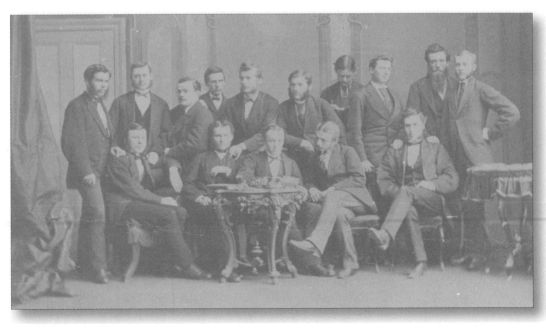

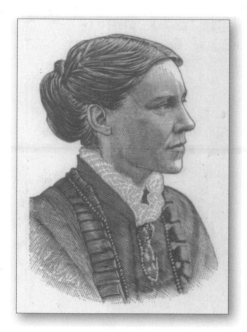

Dr. Jennie Trout was the first woman in Canada to obtain a licence to practise medicine

And she kept on applying. Finally, in 1870, the university relented and allowed Dr. Stowe and another woman, Jennie Trout, to attend. This university session was one of the most unpleasant times in Emily's life. Both the lecturers and the male students did their best to make life as miserable as possible for the two women. Rude drawings were sketched on the classroom walls, and gruesome objects were left on the women's chairs in the hope of frightening them. The staff and students hoped that the women would be so shocked that they would withdraw from the session. But they did not withdraw. Jennie had not taken her training yet but she was sure that she wanted to be a doctor, and Emily knew that she wanted to continue her practice, so the two of them stuck it out and on occasion they fought back. When one of the lecturers continued to encourage the men students' rude behaviour by telling distasteful stories in class, one of the women knew just how to deal with the situation. She went to the lecturer and told him that if he didn't stop this practice, she would tell his wife. The atmosphere in that class improved immediately!

Even after she had attended this session at the University of Toronto Medical School, Emily could not yet get her licence. She still had to take the oral and written examination before the Council of the College of Physicians and Surgeons. This she refused to do for many years, partly because she resented the authority of the Council, which was, of course, made up entirely of men doctors. She also felt that the Council would be reluctant to pass her since she had disturbed their sedate profession with her determination to break into the field, and with the publicity that her success was attracting.

It was not until July 16, 1880, that Emily Stowe finally obtained her licence to practise medicine in Ontario. It was thirteen years since she had graduated from medical school. It had been a long and wearisome battle, but now the Stowe household was filled with celebration.

There were other events for the Stowes to celebrate during these years. Soon after Emily had established her medical practice in Toronto, it expanded so much that she had to move her offices to 111 Church Street. John decided to become a dentist, so Emily again supported him and the family while he trained. In 1878 he graduated and they set up a joint practice at her office on Church Street. The sign outside the door read:

> Emily Stowe, MD – Physician
> John Stowe, LDS – Dentist

The children were greatly influenced by their parents' choices of profession. Since their mother was the only woman practising medicine in the city, indeed, in the entire country for many years, they grew up with a rather different view of life from most other children. Frank used to drive his mother on her rounds in the family's horse and carriage and help deliver the bills.

Augusta learned how good a doctor Emily was from watching her care for her patients. She also learned that there was a desperate need for more women doctors. Great numbers of women came eagerly to Emily for help because they felt they could discuss with her problems that they were too embarrassed to discuss with a man doctor. When men doctors examined their women patients, they had to respect the women's modesty. This meant that women often remained fully clothed for an examination, or were covered in such protective sheets that an accurate diagnosis was very difficult. With a woman doctor, these rules of modesty did not apply.

Augusta also witnessed at first hand her mother's frustration and anger in the attempts to get her licence. She quickly learned that discrimination was very strong against any woman who stepped outside the accepted role of wife and mother. Yet, at the same time as she saw the powerful pressures that her mother had to bear and fight against, Augusta also saw that a woman was fully capable of summoning the strength and determination necessary to win such a fight. She felt that her mother's contribution to medicine was so important that she, too, decided to become a doctor. In 1879, Augusta applied to and was accepted by the Victoria College Medical School.

This pleased Emily and John greatly, and Frank added to their happiness when he decided to become a dentist like his father, and enrolled at the Royal College of Dental Surgeons in Toronto. Their other son, John Howard, thought there were enough doctors in one family, and became a manufacturers' agent.

After all of these triumphs and accomplishments, Emily should have at least been able to sit back and relax a little. Now she could concentrate on her practice and leave the battles against injustice to others. After all, she had done her share in opening up new paths for women.

That may have been what some people thought, but it was not the way Emily felt. During her long struggles for education, for medical training and licensing, and for the respect due to her profession, Emily had realized that she had faced hardships and discrimination mainly because she was a woman. She simply did not have the same rights as a man. This seemed intolerable, and now Emily set out to do something about it.

Young women learning Household Science in the 1800s

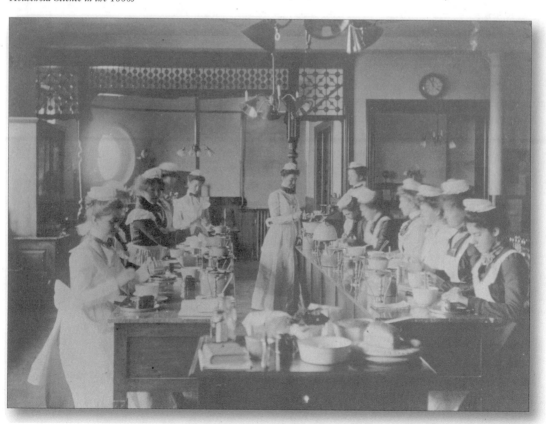

Chapter 6
Women's Rights

It was because she was a woman that Emily had been denied the opportunity to study medicine in Canada, and because of this injustice she had gone to the United States for her medical degree. When she arrived in New York she was painfully aware of the desperate need to improve the lot of women. Emily soon heard about the women in the United States who had been working for a number of years to achieve the same rights as men.

This movement had begun in earnest in 1848 at the Seneca Falls convention arranged by Elizabeth Cady Stanton and Lucretia Mott. Eight years earlier, these two women had realized what woman's position in society really was. They had both been involved for a number of years in the anti-slavery campaign in the United States, working very hard to gain freedom for the slaves. They had known that some people objected to women taking part in the movement and, most of all, to women speaking at meetings. If women were going to help, they should do so quietly and out of sight. But Elizabeth Cady Stanton and Lucretia Mott had both worked with a group of people who welcomed their contribution.

It was not until the World Anti-Slavery Convention in London, England, that they were openly faced with discrimination because they were women. At this convention, in 1840, the male delegates from all over the world refused to have women seated on the convention floor with the men and insisted that they be placed behind a curtain so they could hear the proceedings, but could not speak to the meeting. While a few men fought for the women delegates' right to be full members of the convention, the majority voted against them. The women, including Mrs. Stanton and Mrs. Mott, were seated behind the curtain, and they were angry. After all the work they had done and the knowledge they had

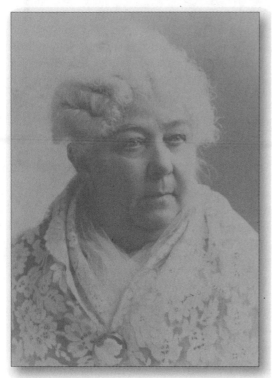
Elizabeth Cady Stanton

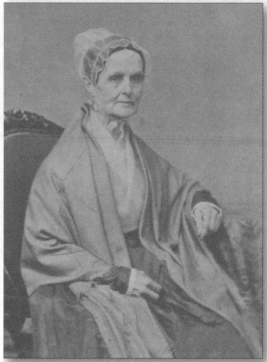
Lucretia Mott

to share, it was disheartening and degrading to be put aside so casually.

The two women talked for long hours about the meaning of such treatment, and after their return to the United States, they continued to question the role that society had given to women. When Mrs. Stanton and Mrs. Mott met again in 1848, they decided to call a convention at Seneca Falls in New York State. The purpose of this meeting was to organize women to fight for equal rights with men.

Twenty years later, the women had petitioned and lectured all over the country. They had fought for the removal of discrimination against women and blacks, and for the abolition of slavery. They had worked and supported their men in the Civil War. They had been praised as heroines and, more often, denounced as troublemakers, but they were little or no further ahead in improving the rights of women. Even so, they were more determined than ever.

When Emily returned to Canada, her licensing problems made her realize that women's situation in Canada was very similar to that of women in the United States. At that time, women in Canada, as in most other countries, had very few legal rights. As Sir William Blackstone, the English jurist, had written: "The husband and wife are one and that one is the husband..." Unmarried women over the age of twenty-one had the same personal and property rights as men, although they did not have the vote. But once a woman married, she lost the right to own property.

What was worse, a wife did not have rights within the family other than the right to be supported by her husband. This meant that she did not even have any say in the guardianship of her children. If her husband wanted to give them up for adoption, send them out to work, educate them or not, the wife had no say. The father could choose the religion of his children and if he died, he could give the children over to a guardian in his will even though their mother was still alive and capable of looking after them.

William Blackstone, 1723–80, the English jurist who wrote the famous Commentaries on the law

Blackstone had said, "Mothers, as such, are entitled to no power, only reverence and respect." If a woman's children were taken away from her by a thoughtless, cruel or drunken husband, reverence and respect did not go very far to help her.

Emily Stowe became so concerned over women's lack of rights that soon after she returned to Canada, she began travelling all over southern Ontario giving talks to women, even while she carried on a full medical practice and cared for her family. She felt it was most important that women should understand how many rights they did not have. Many women came to these talks to hear what she had to say. This also gave them the chance to talk to a woman doctor about the ailments and problems that they were too modest to take to a man doctor. Emily used these discussions to talk about many topics, such as education for women. She thought that girls should have the same education as boys. Emily discussed the position of women, pointing out the injustices and arguing that women could do a lot of good if their rights were improved.

In 1876, she went to Cleveland to attend a meeting of the American Society for the Advancement of Women. There she met a group of people who had organized themselves to fight the inequality of women. She returned to Toronto convinced that Canadian women, too, should unite to improve their status.

Women often did the same work as men but did not have the same rights.

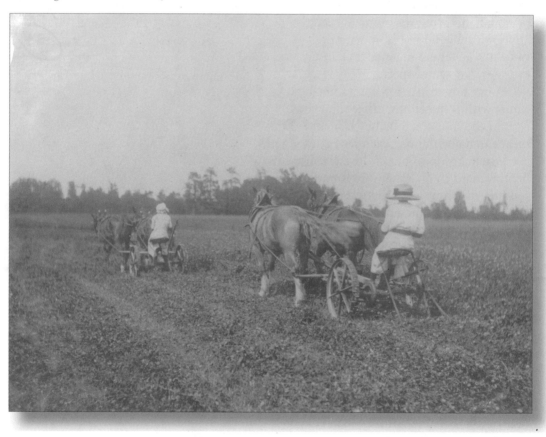

Chapter 7
The Suffrage Movement

In Toronto Emily talked with many of her women friends about women's rights, and she found a good deal of support. So, in November, 1876, Emily Stowe founded the first Canadian women's organization to fight for equal rights for women. Among its first members were Mrs. Sarah Ann Curzon, Miss Helen Archibald, Mrs. D. McEwan, Mrs. Anna Parker and Miss Jenny Gray. Out of all the appropriate names that might have been chosen for this group, the members decided to call it the Toronto Women's Literary Club. This may seem an odd choice for an organization they hoped would be able to make vast changes in legal and social systems. But the members of the club judged, and rightly so, that society was not yet ready for an open attack on its standards. This innocent-sounding name allowed them to discuss the problems that they faced without annoying the people who would vigorously oppose the reforms they wanted.

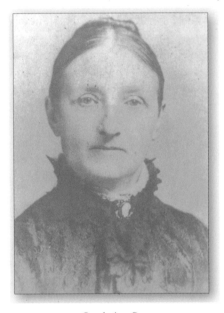

Sarah Ann Curzon

The Toronto Women's Literary Club met once a week, on Thursdays, at different members' homes. They talked about a broad range of subjects, and each woman took a turn at speaking on a topic. One evening Miss Archibald spoke about "The Enfranchisement of Women," and another time Emily talked about the need for better education for girls. They discussed politics and health; they looked at the economic and working conditions of women; and they accomplished a fair bit.

Under Emily's leadership, the women managed to obtain better sanitary arrangements for women who worked in factories. Until the Literary Club started to raise a few questions, factory women did not even have separate washrooms from the men. When Emily and her friends had helped to improve the conditions for women in factories, they turned their attention to store clerks. At that time, clerks usually worked a twelve-hour day, six days a week. During that long day, they had only a short lunch hour and spent the rest of the time on their feet. The Literary Club members agitated and campaigned until finally they persuaded the store owners to provide seats for the clerks.

One of the members, Mrs. Sarah Ann Curzon, was particularly helpful in the work of the Toronto Literary Club. She became associate editor of a Toronto weekly, *Canada Citizen*, and used her column to support the women's ideas and, later, to support women's suffrage.

In 1881, Emily and a few other members of the club formed a deputation to the provincial government to ask for the vote for women. The following year they had a small success. The Ontario Legislature passed a law that permitted unmarried women to vote on municipal bylaws if they had the necessary property qualification. Two years later, unmarried women were granted full voting rights in municipal elections. Since one of Emily's great concerns was for higher education for women, the club sent a petition to the legislature in 1882, asking that women be admitted to the University of Toronto. In 1884, they won that request and women students began their studies at the university with the 1886-87 session.

In the meantime, Emily and the members of the Toronto Women's Literary Club decided that they had disguised their true goals long enough. On March 9, 1883, at a meeting at Toronto City Hall, the club formally reorganized itself and took the new name, Toronto Women's Suffrage Association. Its goal was equal suffrage for women.

The women came very close to achieving this goal almost immediately, for it was at this time that the Prime Minister, Sir John A. Macdonald, introduced a bill in Parliament proposing uniform federal enfranchisement. However, there was such an uproar and so many were against the inclusion of women, that the Prime Minister was forced to drop that clause from the bill. The women's movement might be underway, but Emily Stowe and her supporters still had to face a great deal of opposition.

But Emily was not just concerned about the vote for women. She had been annoyed and angry about all the unnec-

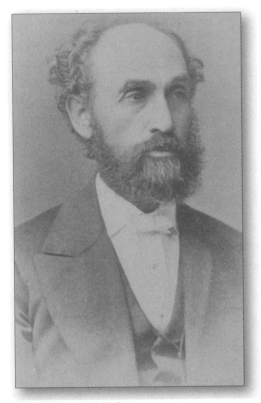
Dr. Samuel Sobiestic Nelles

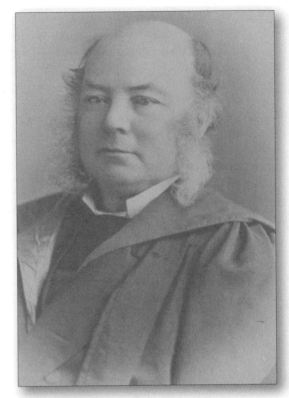
Dr. Michael Barrett

essary difficulties she had had to face to get her medical degree. Now she was determined to try to remove the obstacles and make it easier for other women to get medical training. Even though her daughter Augusta had been accepted by the Victoria College Medical School, this had been due largely to Emily's influence and to the Stowe family's long-standing friendship with the Nelles family in Mount Pleasant. Dr. William Nelles's brother, Dr. Samuel Sobiestic Nelles, was principal of Victoria College and he had been sympathetic to Augusta's desire to become a doctor.

But this did not make it easier for other women who did not have the same relatives and friends. So Emily lectured and campaigned and persuaded. A number of people were sympathetic to her arguments, particularly Dr. Michael Barrett, Professor of Physiology at the University of Toronto. He felt Emily was right that women should be able to train as doctors, but he thought it would be better if the women took their training separately from the men. So he suggested that a special medical college for women should be opened.

On June 13, 1883, the Toronto Women's Suffrage Association held a public meeting in Shaftesbury Hall to discuss the idea of a women's medical college. Many influential people attended, such as Mr. James Beatty, MP, Dr. James Carlyle, and Professor Thomas Kirkland from the Normal School. The Hon. Justice Patterson chaired the meeting and, after much discussion, Mr. Beatty proposed a motion that a medical college for women should be provided. The motion met with the approval of the meeting and Dr. Barrett spoke to the group about his plans for such a college.

With so many powerful people involved and with so much enthusiasm for the idea, it did not take long to put the plan

The house at 289 Sumach Street where the Ontario Medical College for Women first opened

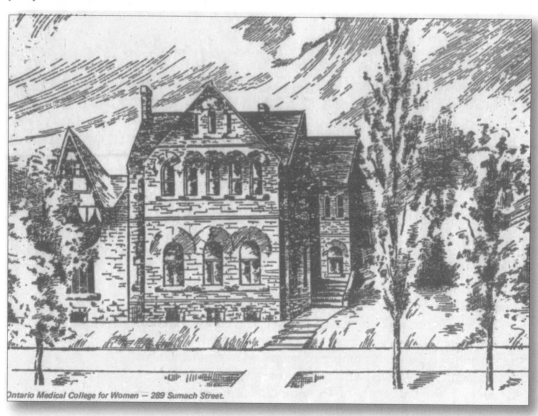

Ontario Medical College for Women — 289 Sumach Street.

into action. On October 1, that same year, the Ontario Medical College for Women opened its doors. Emily was delighted because once again she had helped make one of her happiest dreams become a reality.

The college originally started out in a rented building on 289 Sumach Street in Toronto. But by 1890 it had outgrown these quarters and moved to its own building on Sackville Street. Here it also opened clinics so that women patients could be treated by women physicians. The Ontario Medical College for Women finally closed its doors in 1906 when the University of Toronto at last agreed to accept women in its medical classes. The clinics were still kept open and eventually became Women's College Hospital, which is now part of Sunnybrook and Women's College Health Sciences Centre.

The original Women's College Hospital on Rusholme Road, Toronto

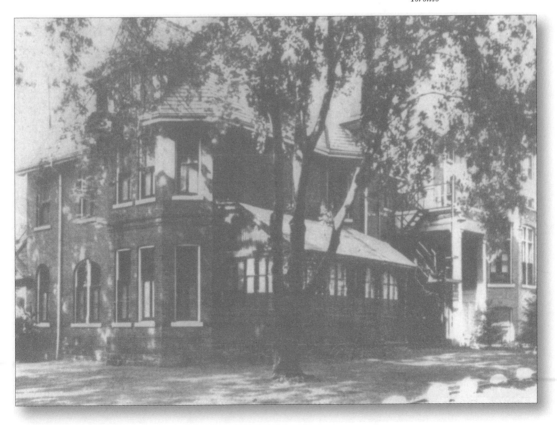

Chapter 8
The Struggle for the Vote

In spite of their success in establishing the Ontario Medical College for Women, the Suffrage Association was not getting very far in its struggle to obtain the vote for women. The members regularly sent petitions and deputations of women, usually led by Emily, to the provincial and municipal governments. But the answer was always the same; their requests were denied.

The members had been working very hard with little to show for their time and dedication, and gradually the enthusiasm was going out of the movement. But Emily never lost her desire to see improvements in the rights of women. She realized that many of the members had become discouraged when all their work and effort so often came to nothing, but she also knew that women would never be able to improve society without the right to vote. And they would never get the right if they didn't continue to fight for it. So Emily renewed her efforts and, at a meeting at her home early in 1889, she and a group of friends decided to invite Dr. Anna Howard Shaw to come to Toronto to speak.

Dr. Shaw was a famous American suffragist who was well-known as a lively speaker. On January 31, she spoke to a packed house with such power and persuasion that members of the audience were thoroughly convinced of the need to keep working for their cause. In the days following Dr. Shaw's speech, a number of meetings were held and again Emily spoke about issues of concern to women. As a result, the Dominion Women's Enfranchisement Association was formed, with Dr. Emily Stowe as the president. Once again petitions began to flow into the legislature and deputations arrived regularly to try to persuade Attorney-General Mowat and his party to give women the vote.

On February 8, 1889, Mayor Clarke of Toronto introduced a delegation from the Association and the Women's Christian Temperance Union to the Ontario Legislature. Emily spoke on behalf of the group and their request for women's rights:

We do as educated citizens, as moral and loving women, desire to be placed in a position to impress directly our thoughts upon our nation and times.

She also answered one of the common arguments against giving women the vote. Women, it was often stated, were not intelligent enough to be able to use the vote wisely even if they had it. Emily countered:

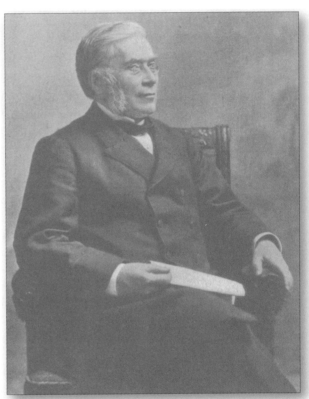

If the women of our country are not all prepared to use the newly imposed responsibility intelligently, neither are men prepared to use it intelligently. Of this I am certain, that the women of our country desire to use it only for their country's good.

The women were at the legislature to support a bill put before the house by John Waters. The bill did not ask a great deal, only that widows and spinsters be given the right to vote in provincial elections. While the members

Sir Oliver Mowat

of the delegation would rather have had a bill asking for the vote for all women, they felt this one was a step in the right direction and they were prepared to support it. The bill, however, was defeated.

The suffragists had found an ardent supporter of their cause in John Waters. He was a Liberal member of the Ontario Legislature who became involved in the struggle for women's right to vote provincially. Between 1885 and 1893, he brought numerous bills before the legislature. None of them was successful, but some progress was made. The first of these bills was greeted with hoots of laughter and indignation, but as Waters continued to introduce measures and as the women continued to petition, the members of the legislature began to treat the matter more seriously. This did not mean there were any changes in the law, but it did show that the women's proposals were no longer being dismissed as ridiculous.

However, there were still many arguments against granting votes to women. Some of these were very silly, such as the argument that women were not as mentally capable as men and so would not vote wisely. But the greatest fear was that giving women the vote would destroy the harmony of the home. Some people believed that a family would not be able to survive the strain if a husband and wife voted for different candidates. Many said that women already had the power of the vote because they could influence, with loving persuasion, the man who had the right to vote. Emily quickly pointed out that many women did not have such influence over their husbands, and others did not have a husband to influence.

Another argument was that the right to vote carried with it the responsibility of fighting for one's country, and women did not do this. And even if women were given the vote, they wouldn't use it and so there was no point in giving it to them. Some said that allowing women to vote was against the teachings of the Bible.

The suffragists had answers for all these arguments as well as counterarguments why women should have the vote. They carefully put together evidence to show that large numbers of men never used the vote that was rightfully theirs, and this did not mean these men lost their right to vote. They pointed out that women paid taxes and, therefore, had a right to help shape the laws. If they did not, it was taxation without representation and revolutions had been started over just that issue. The women felt that because they were concerned with their families and homes, they would have special influence on moral questions and they could help a great deal in matters of education and health. Some claimed that if women had the power of the vote, there would be no more war. So far, this has not proved to be true.

Emily wrote many letters to newspapers and government officials. She continued her speaking engagements, explaining and justifying the women's demands. The Association asked Dr. Shaw to return to Toronto to speak and, in December, 1889, they invited another famous American suffragist, Susan B. Anthony. Miss Anthony was one of the leaders of the movement in the United States and her speech in the United States and her speech in Toronto excited and encouraged the large audience. Susan was to become a good friend of Emily and her daughter and often returned to Toronto to visit with them. On those visits they would have long and lively discussions about the status of women in both countries, and about how much work still had to be done.

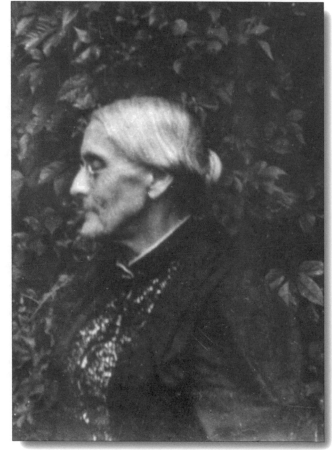

Susan B. Anthony

By 1890, the Canadian suffragists decided the time had come to co-ordinate the efforts of all the women's groups across the country. On June 12 and 13, they held the first Dominion Conference. It was attended by representatives from across Canada and many from the United States. One of the representatives was Dr. Stowe's sister, Dr. Hannah Kimball. Hannah and another sister, Ella, had followed in Emily's footsteps and had both become doctors. They practised in the United States.

The Dominion Conference was a great success. All around the hall where the meetings were held were hung signs that the women had made. "Canada's Daughters Should be Free," said one, and another read, "Women Are Half the People." Talks were given by a number of the delegates, including one on the "History of the Women's Suffrage Movement in

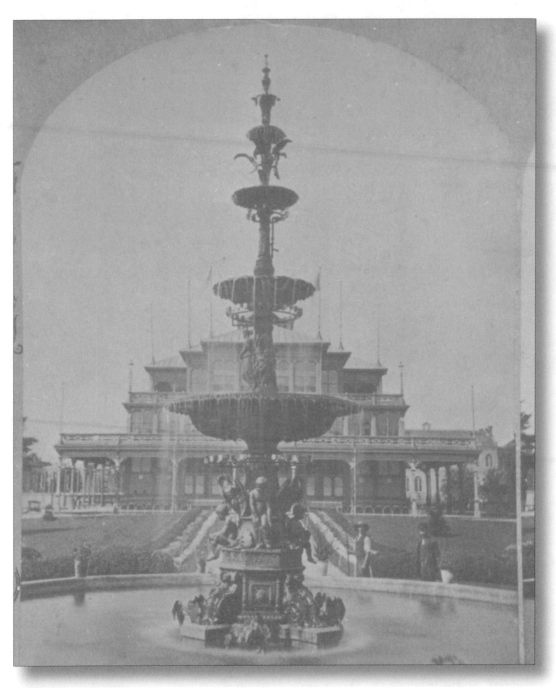

The Pavilion at Allan Gardens in Toronto

Canada." Emily was given credit for starting the movement and for being the force that kept it going. Both the Canadian and American delegates felt that Emily's contribution to the suffrage movement was outstanding and deserved recognition so they re-elected her president of the Association. Emily was honoured, but she realized that the fight was far from over. There was much more to do and greater support was needed before they would be successful.

Sometimes it seemed that the women were too serious, but in spite of many setbacks and defeats, they could still use humour to make their points. In 1896 they organized a mock parliament at the Pavilion, in what is now Allan Gardens in Toronto. Here the women all played the roles of various members of the legislature, just as if women had always been in power. They received a delegation of men who were seeking the right to vote. Emily played the part of the Attorney-General, Sir Oliver Mowat, and her daughter, Augusta, was the Minister of Crown Lands.

The men in the delegation asked humbly to be granted the basic right of any citizen, the right to vote. The women legislators, with clever humour, imitated the responses that they had received so often. They pointed out that giving men the vote would mean that soon men would be wanting to wear women's clothes and be admitted to women's professions and this would disrupt society. Men were designed to do the heavy work and should leave the running of the country to the more capable women. On top of this, the mock parliament ruled that giving men the right to vote would be against the teachings of the Scriptures. So the men's request was refused. The mock parliament was very successful and the local newspapers gave it full coverage. The suffragists' cause gained very favourable and much needed publicity.

Chapter 9
The Torch Is Passed

In 1891, Emily suffered a deep personal loss with the death of her husband, John. Although not a great deal is known about John Stowe, he played a very important role throughout Emily's struggles. While many men were firmly opposed to women having a career or the vote and some even went to great lengths to stop women getting them, John Stowe encouraged his wife in all her efforts. Just as Emily had helped him during his illness and in his career, so he stood by her and helped her in her career and campaigns. He was a constant source of strength for Emily as she struggled time after time to gain greater opportunities for women.

Stowe Island on Lake Joseph

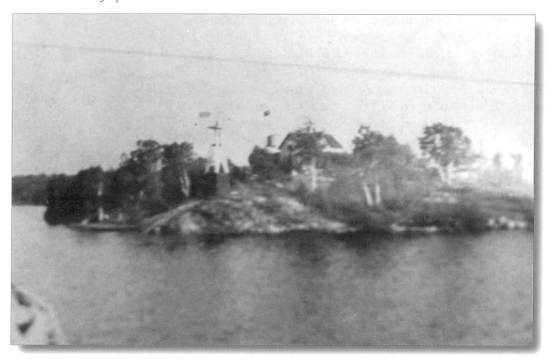

Chapter 10
Augusta the Doctor

One reason for Emily's continued influence was that after her death, another woman stepped forward to fill her shoes and provide a vital and strong leadership for the suffrage movement. That woman was Dr. Augusta Stowe-Gullen, Emily's daughter.

Augusta had been working alongside her mother for many years as Emily tried to convince Canadian men and women of the need to give women the vote. She learned a good deal from Emily about organizing groups and speaking to audiences, large and small, and rapidly became as powerful a force as Emily in the struggle for women's rights. But Augusta's first step in her mother's footsteps had been taken much earlier.

By 1878 she had decided to become a doctor, and promptly began preparations to take the matriculation examinations that had to be passed by every student entering medical school. It is a bit surprising that Augusta, who was to be such a successful doctor, failed her maths the first time she tried the exams. But in 1879, she passed and was admitted to the Victoria College Medical School.

By this time there was a good deal of interest in allowing women to become doctors. Emily Stowe and Jennie Trout had proven to even the most doubtful that women could stand the rigours of the profession. Queen's University in Kingston was the first to give women a chance at a medical career. They offered a series of summer courses so that the women students could train separately from the men. Many people still felt that having men and women students in the same class, studying the human body together, was immodest and quite unacceptable. In 1881, the women students were finally admitted to the full-time course, but the summer school plan meant it took much longer to complete the course. Therefore, Queen's did not graduate its first women doctors till 1884.

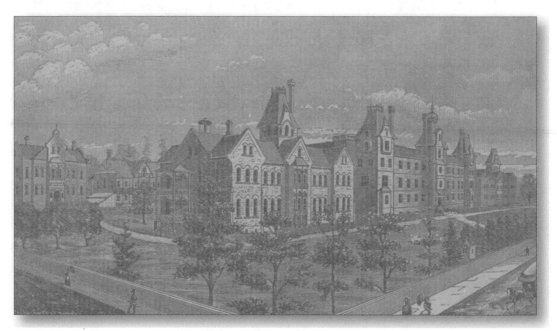

Toronto General Hospital, where Augusta did her internship

Augusta was not caught in this confusion of courses at Queen's University because she had decided to try for admission at the medical school at Victoria College. One very important reason for this decision was that Emily did not approve of the summer course system at Queen's. Examining and dissecting animal tissue in the heat of the summer months would be most unpleasant. Emily also felt that learning medicine through summer courses would take too long.

While Augusta was studying at Victoria College, the medical students had their classes at the Toronto School of Medicine, just across the street from the Toronto General Hospital. It was there that Augusta interned from 1879 to 1883. It was very convenient for Augusta since she could live at home, and that may have been another reason for her choosing Victoria College.

Augusta knew that life had not been very pleasant for Emily when she had taken just one session at the University of Toronto Medical School, and it was not much easier for Augusta. She said once, when describing her medical training,

The first pioneer woman to study medicine in Canada, had not a pathway strewn with roses.

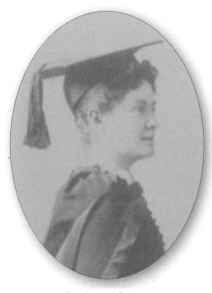
Dr. Augusta Stowe

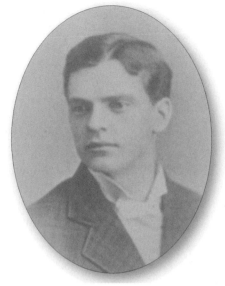
Dr. John Gullen

As the only woman student in the class, she was often the victim of mean jokes and rude behaviour, like her mother before her. This treatment affected her very deeply.

She would cry all the way from the college to her home, vowing she would never return. Her mother would put her loving arms around her, comforting and counselling her. Even then she would cry herself to sleep. Every day her father would accompany her to and from school. Students and some of the professors took a delight in insulting drawings and diagrams on the blackboard and on her desk. In the dissecting room it was even worse.

But Augusta was a fighter, like her mother, and there was a limit to what she would take. One day, tired of this treatment,

...with just anger and scorn, she stepped back, straightened up, and with hands on hips, gave the ring leader a scathing dressing down for such degrading and mortifying remarks...Afterwards this same student stood up and defended her on all occasions.

She never revealed the name of that student.

In 1883 when Augusta graduated, she was the first woman to do so from a Canadian medical school. This was a most suitable honour for the daughter of the first Canadian woman doctor, and Emily was justifiably proud. As Augusta accepted her diploma at the graduation ceremonies, "the entire audience sprang to its feet and cheered vociferously for several minutes."

Augusta had triumphed. She had not only earned her medical degree, but she had also so convinced her fellow students of her dedication and determination that they changed their attitudes towards this woman who wanted to be a doctor. So strongly did she influence one classmate that he asked her to marry him. Shortly after their graduation, Dr. Augusta Stowe and Dr. John Benjamin Gullen were married on May 23, at 7:30 pm in a beautiful wedding ceremony at the Metropolitan

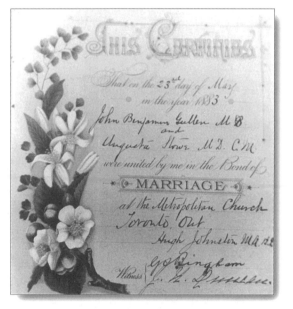

John and Augusta's marriage certificate, the first for two Canadian doctors

Church in Toronto. Large crowds were on hand to see Augusta arrive at the church with her father. She was dressed in traditional white, with a veil and a wreath of orange blossoms. After the marriage ceremony, many friends were invited to the Stowe home for the wedding reception.

This wedding was another first for Augusta as it was the first marriage between two Canadian doctors. Their honeymoon was as unusual as their wedding. Instead of taking a relaxing holiday, the two of them went to New York to take a postgraduate course in children's diseases.

Shortly after Augusta and John returned from New York, Augusta was appointed Demonstrator of Anatomy at the newly formed Ontario Medical College for Women. At the beginning she was the only woman on the staff. Augusta was to remain deeply committed to the college until it finally closed its doors in 1906 when the University of Toronto Medical School agreed to take women students. Before that time, however, she went on to become Professor of Diseases of Children; later she served as president of the Alumnae Association and eventually was appointed a director of the College.

Despite her obvious commitment to the welfare of the Ontario Medical College for Women, Augusta did not confine her medical knowledge to this one area. While she was involved with the Medical College, she also ran a private practice at her home on Spadina Avenue, which she and John had purchased in 1889.

Even this workload was not enough for Augusta. Like her mother, she possessed boundless energy and she became involved with Western Hospital, partly because her husband was one of the founders. Augusta worked closely with John and even before the hospital was fully open, she was the doctor who delivered its first baby on November 1, 1896. Because the hospital had just started and was in need of many items, Augusta organized the doctors' wives into the Women's Board of Western Hospital. It was the endless efforts of this group that provided the hospital with necessary linen, much of its equipment and, eventually, the nurses' residence. Augusta served as president of the Women's Board until 1928, and when she retired, the members of the Board showed their appreciation for all she had done by presenting her with a beautiful silver tea service.

Toronto Western Hospital

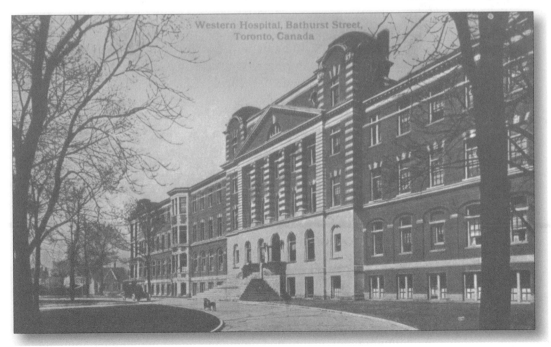

Chapter 11
Augusta the Suffragist

Augusta's interests did not only lie in the field of medicine. Like her mother, she had suffered from discrimination because she had chosen to pursue a career outside the role of wife and mother. For many years she had worked with her mother in the suffrage movement and she felt that definite steps had to be taken to improve the situation of women in Canada. But she did not want a total revolution, for there were some aspects of being a woman that Augusta liked very much. She was particularly fond of clothes and was always beautifully dressed in elaborate long dresses cinched tightly at the waist. This fashion was very hard on women. The long skirts were constantly in the way, they picked up dirt and dust everywhere, and they made walking very difficult. It was almost impossible to climb stairs without at least one hand free to lift the skirt. It would be dangerous for a woman to climb the stairs carrying a baby and an oil lamp. The tight corsets that made a woman's waist so tiny squeezed the internal organs and made it difficult to breathe. This often caused indigestion and also explained why women were inclined to faint. The whole outfit, created from layer upon layer of outer and undergarments, was incredibly hot and heavy.

As far back as 1851, Elizabeth Smith Miller had introduced a much more sensible outfit in the United States.

Instead of fitting snugly, their waists were comfortably loose, and their skirts, instead of sweeping the streets according to respectable fashion, ended just below their knees. Under the skirts they wore long pantaloons, ballooning out very full, then gathered closely at the ankles, where they ended in a short ruffle.

A stylish outfit from the 1890s

This became known as the bloomer costume because a woman named Amelia Bloomer championed the outfit in her feminist paper, *The Lily*. She also gave talks to women about the wisdom of abandoning the more restrictive fashion in favour of this outfit which was suitably modest, but gave the wearer complete freedom of movement. The enthusiasm for this outfit did not last long as the few women who wore it were laughed at. Small boys jeered at them on the streets,

Heigh! ho!
Thro' sleet and snow,
Mrs. Bloomer's all the go.
Twenty tailors take the
 stitches,
Plenty of women wear the
 breeches,
Heigh! Ho!
Carrion crow.

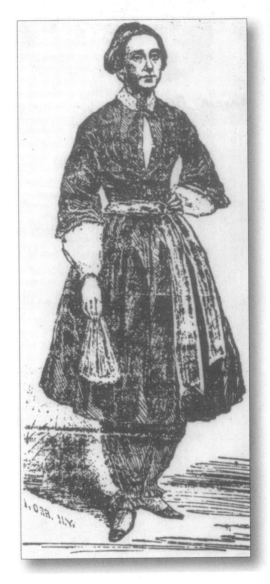

Amelia Bloomer in the costume she made famous

Finally, the women gave in and went back to wearing long heavy skirts and corsets, knowing that they were losing a good deal.

Although she was a doctor and must have realized the health hazards involved, Augusta still dressed fashionably. She was an impressive figure in her long, well-styled dresses, her beautiful hair piled high on her head and topped with a fashionable hat. She did once don the bloomer costume, but that was only to prove a point. Dressed in bloomers, jacket and

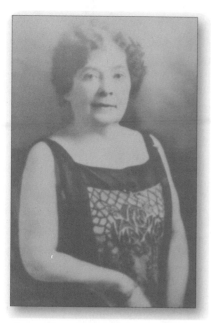

Augusta Stowe-Gullen

cap, she rode a bicycle down Yonge Street to demonstrate that women had the right to do so.

Augusta may have liked to wear elaborate clothes and to be thought attractive, but she did not like the limits placed on rights for women and the lack of equality with men. She was involved from the beginning with the Toronto Women's Literary Club and one time gave a talk to the members about the numerous women throughout history who had been capable and prudent rulers.

While she worked ceaselessly with her mother in the campaign for women's suffrage, Augusta did not confine her energies to the Suffrage Club. She was very concerned that girls should have the same opportunity as boys for a full education because, she said, "If education be commendable or necessary for man it is equally so for woman." So in 1892, Augusta ran in the municipal election for the position of school trustee in Ward 4. She was successful and was one of three women elected to the Toronto School Board that year. She served on the board till 1896, and during those four years she was a champion of women teachers. At one point, the board decided to cut expenses by lowering the salaries of women principals. Men principals' salaries were not, of course, to be cut. Augusta fought the proposal and was successful in defeating it.

After her mother's death, Augusta became president of the Dominion Women's Enfranchisement Association. Renewed enthusiasm flowed through the organization and delegations once again began to appear at the legislature. In 1905 the Liberal Party was defeated and the Conservatives came to power under the leadership of Premier J.P. Whitney. Augusta led her Association, along with members of the Women's Christian Temperance Union, in an attempt to get the municipal franchise for married women. Seventy-two petitions from cities and towns in Ontario were submitted in favour of extending the franchise. But Premier Whitney would not support a change.

James P. Whitney

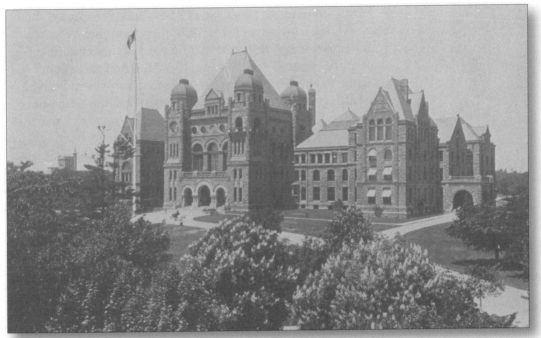

The new Ontario Parliament Buildings, Queen's Park, where the suffragists presented their petitions in 1909

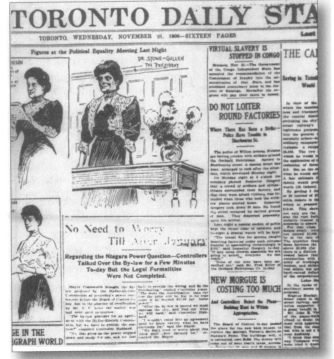

From the Toronto Daily Star, *November 21, 1906*

Disappointed but determined, the women continued their efforts. Under Augusta's leadership, the Dominion Women's Enfranchisement Association continued to campaign for support of the franchise for women. In 1907, the DWEA changed its name to the Canadian Suffrage Association which was less awkward for the press and public. Under this new name they redoubled their efforts.

By 1909, they had organized a huge delegation to the provincial legislature. On March 24, one thousand people descended upon the Parliament Buildings, overflowing the reception room and corridors. They represented fourteen different organizations and they brought with them a petition requesting full suffrage for women in Ontario. It had been signed by one hundred thousand people. The effect of so large a delegation should have been overwhelming. Dr. Augusta Stowe-Gullen presented the petition to Premier Whitney and was one of a number of men and women who spoke on behalf of the organizations they represented. The Premier, however, was not impressed and would not change his stand. It is hard to believe that the Premier, elected by the people, would refuse even to consider their demands in the face of such large and consistent support among the people for full suffrage for women.

In 1911 another delegation, this one much smaller, again approached Premier Whitney. Two hundred women were there, each wearing a yellow daffodil because yellow was the adopted colour of the suffrage movement. Again Augusta was one of the speakers, but again the suffrage bill they were supporting was defeated.

This was the year that Augusta stepped down as the president of the Canadian Suffrage Association. She was not giving up her fight for equal rights and the vote for women, but she felt it was time for a new leader to stimulate the efforts of the Association. She would continue her involvement in other ways. A banquet was held to honour Augusta on her retirement from the presidency and many tributes were paid to her for her contributions to the women's cause. One highlight of the dinner was the presence of Mrs. Emmeline Pankhurst, the famous English suffragette, who was in Canada on a speaking tour.

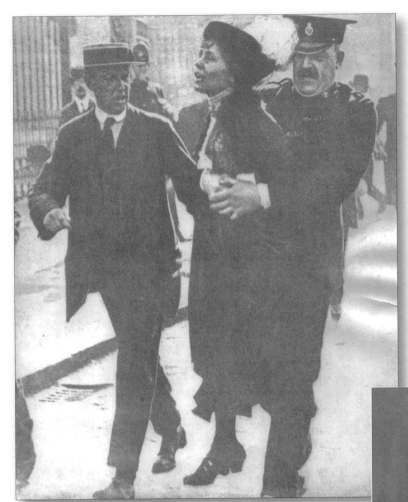

Augusta remained as the honorary president of the Suffrage Association and became vice-president of the National Council of Women. This was a very powerful organization founded in 1893 by Lady Aberdeen, wife of the governor-general. The National Council of Women was the Canadian branch of the International Council of Women. Early in the 1900s this group decided to support the suffrage movement and added worldwide support to the cause.

Lady Aberdeen

Augusta the Suffragist

Since 1904, Augusta had been the chairwoman of the NCW Standing Committee on Suffrage and Rights of Citizenship, a position she held until 1921 when she was sixty-four years old. As well, in 1910, Augusta had been appointed to the University of Toronto Senate as the medical profession representative. It is ironic that she should receive such an appointment when it was an earlier senate from the same university that had denied her mother the right to study medicine and had fought so hard against allowing women into the University of Toronto Medical School. It must have been with a great deal of satisfaction that Augusta accepted the appointment.

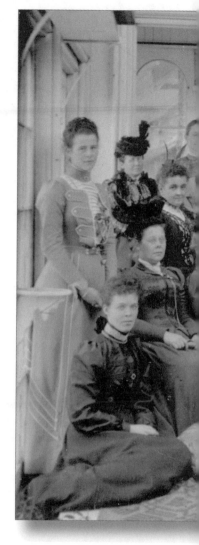

While serving actively on these different committees, Augusta also found time to travel. And she travelled all over. In 1895 she had gone to Europe and seen the beautiful cities of Geneva, Rome and Florence. To support the women's movement, she travelled to New Orleans, New York, Chicago, Winnipeg and throughout Ontario, giving lectures on the need to improve the status of women and the need for child labour laws.

Even these demanding commitments were not enough for her. She served as vice-president of the Ontario Social Service Council and was an active member of the University Women's Club and the Women's Art Association. At the same time, she continued her private medical practice from the office in her home on Spadina Avenue. So greatly did Canada benefit from her dedication in so many fields that in 1935 she was awarded the King's Medal.

Augusta the Suffragist

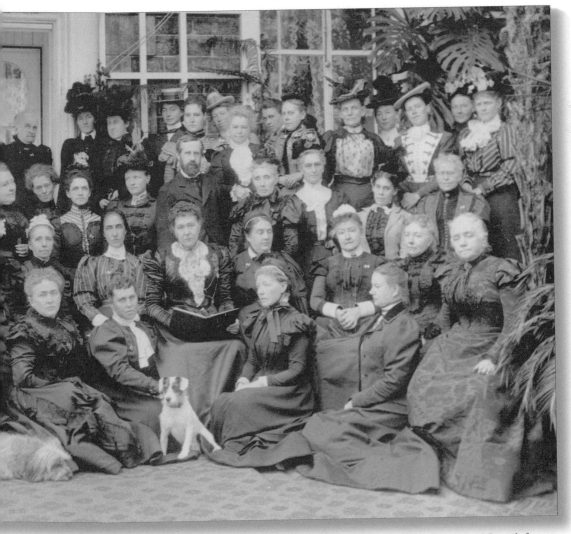

The National Council of Women at Rideau Hall, Ottawa. Lady Aberdeen, the founder, is in the centre.

Augusta died in Toronto in September, 1943, one year before her husband, John. Just a few months earlier, the two of them had happily celebrated the sixtieth anniversary of their graduation and their wedding.

She had led a full, active life and, like her mother, Augusta was committed to getting the vote for women and to improving their status in Canada. Unlike her mother, she lived to see women given the right to vote.

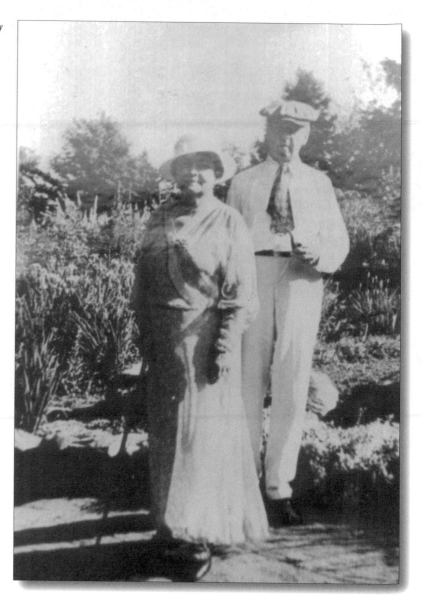

Augusta and John occasionally found time to relax in Muskoka

Epilogue

O n April 12, 1917, royal assent was given to the bill granting full suffrage to the women of Ontario. The Western Provinces had already granted women the right to vote (Manitoba, Saskatchewan and Alberta in 1916, and British Columbia on April 5, 1917). The Ontario Liberal Party had, at last, come out officially in support of women's suffrage. With an election coming up, the Conservatives, led by Premier William Hearst, changed their stand and supported the bills giving women the right to vote in provincial and municipal elections. Premier Hearst claimed that he was sure most women still did not want the right to vote, but women had made so great a contribution to the Canadian war effort that they had earned the right to vote. He did not, however, acknowledge that women had been contributing to Canadian life since the first settlers had arrived and that the denial of the vote to women had been unjust and discriminatory from the beginning.

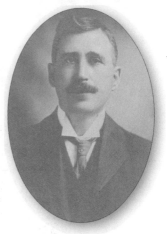

William H. Hearst

In 1906 the University of Toronto had finally accepted women students in its Medical School. By that time the Ontario Medical College for Women had already graduated more than one hundred women doctors. Many of these were outstanding physicians in their chosen fields and contributed to the advancement of medicine all over the world.

Women's rights, both to vote and to become doctors, were made possible by the work of Dr. Emily Howard Stowe and her daughter, Dr. Augusta Stowe-Gullen. Both these women had devoted their lives to improving the status of women in Canada. Each had fought with determination and persistence to gain for women the right to vote and to have a say in the laws and regulations that affected their lives as well as the lives of men. Both Emily and Augusta had proved beyond a shadow of a doubt that women had much to contribute to Canadian

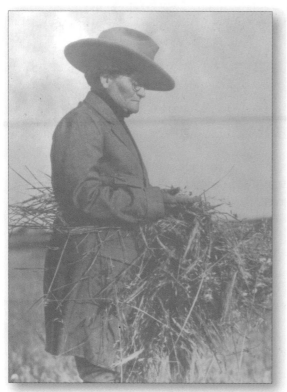

E. Cora Hind

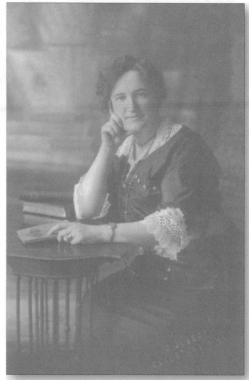

Nellie McClung

society. In particular, they had proved that women were necessary and important in the field of medicine.

They were two very unusual people for their time who inspired many others to join in the fight and support their cause. A number of other women devoted themselves to improving the lives of Canadian women in many ways. Such women as Emily Murphy, Nellie McClung, Clara Brett Martin and E. Cora Hind had helped to change the laws and restrictions that confined women. But these women, like Emily Stowe and Augusta Stowe-Gullen, had to fight against the strong opinions most Canadians held that a woman's place was

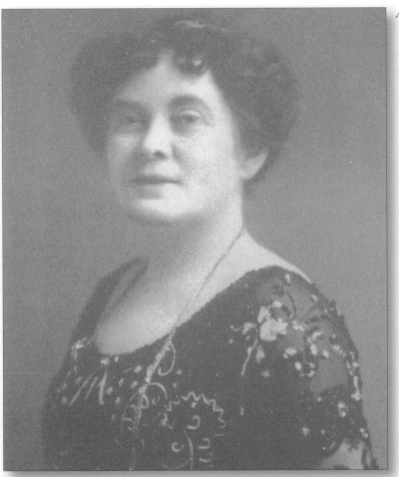

in the home. They had to show by their own experiences that going out of the home to pursue a career or to become involved in politics was not immoral and immodest. To win their battles, they had to prove that women could be good wives and mothers as well as good citizens. They had to prove that women had the strength, intelligence and determination to succeed. And succeed they did.

Emily Stowe

1831 Born on May 1 in Norwich, Ontario

1854 Graduates from the Normal School for Upper Canada and becomes first woman principal in Canada

1856 Marries John Stowe

1867 Graduates from New York Medical College for Women; Sets up practice in Toronto

1870 Attends classes at University of Toronto Medical School

1876 Attends a meeting in Cleveland of the American Society for the Advancement of Women; Founds the Toronto Women's Literary Club

1879 Daughter Augusta enters Victoria College Medical School

1880 Receives licence to practise medicine in Ontario

1883 Literary Club is renamed Toronto Women's Suffrage Association; Ontario Medical College for Women is opened; Augusta graduates from medical school and marries Dr. John Gullen

1889 Becomes President of the Dominion Women's Enfranchisement Association; Addresses the Ontario Legislature regarding women's rights

1891 John Stowe dies

1892 Augusta is elected school trustee for the Toronto School Board

1893 Retires from the medical profession

1896 Holds mock parliament in Toronto

1903 Dies on April 30 in Toronto